An Hour to Begin

Short Stories in Fiction and Nonfiction

Tabitha Young

authorHOUSE®

AuthorHouse™
1663 Liberty Drive
Bloomington, IN 47403
www.authorhouse.com
Phone: 1 (800) 839-8640

Published by AuthorHouse   05/31/2019

ISBN: 978-1-7283-1240-8 (sc)
ISBN: 978-1-7283 1239 2 (e)

Print information available on the last page.

This book is printed on acid-free paper.

Contents

1. Thicker than Water...1

2. The Snail and the Pink Watch 3

3. Separate and Friendly-Is it Possible? : Part 1 5

4. Separate and Friendly: Part 2 7

5. Where Cats Bow..9

6. Three Dogs Down 10

7. Finding a Bubbling Creek 11

8. What is Schizoaffective? 14

9. Had to be the One...25

10. The Lighthouse Keeper 26

11. Her Story...28

12. Billy Sunshine 29

13. How the Porcupine Got It's Quills 31

14. Description of a Superhero...32

15. "An Hour to Begin" 33

16. Donovan and the Three Dogs..35

17. A Mothers Smile...36

18. Making a Name 40

19. Heaven on the Mountaintop..42

20. Domino Effect- 44

About The Author 49

This short story series is dedicated to my first best friend Crystal Combs. I really hope we meet again one day and I wish her well. I know the emotion is mutual. Playing doll house as children is fun and got me to really join creativity and to imagine.

Thicker than Water

Marty and Matthew McClelland are twin brothers. They do not finish each other's sentences but in a way that is how they put forth actions. In almost a fantasy ending they get what they want even when well, let me tell you what happened.

"Break a leg on that test today boys," says Able Sable.

Today Matthew is taking a test for a job like Marty is the younger twin.

Matthew a studious party- prepared ahead of time and landed a cool B+. Marty although unprepared made an A finish. Feeling insecure, Matthew, upon exiting, drops his no. 2 pencil on the table which was borrowed and switches the test with his brothers. They have the same handwriting.

Later, Marty shows up after a little drink at a party where he meets up with Janella- the so-called love of his life. She sways her hips to the music blaring and walks up to Marty.

"Hey, you wanna dance?" Janella says.

"Nope, Monica. Not right now. I been thinking about my Mom.

"You should go Marty/' says Janella.

With a slip of his hand across gently Janella' face he kisses her on the lips and walks out.

A few minutes later he finds himself at Salome Vasquez McClelland's tombstone.

"Hi. You know goodbye was easier for Matthew, Able Sable and Daddy. I know you possibly cannot hear me but I am so angry you left me!

You taught me everything even though you were a woman- Mommy! But I forgive you, only you.

He sings a Christina Aguilera song to himself: ((It seems the storm has passed. Through it all, no one knew. That all the tears in heaven would bring me back to you, oh. Christina Aguilera was his mom's favorite in the past.

Also, he goes home. He does not speak to anyone, not even ((Uncle"
Able Sable.

"Where did you learn to turn your back on an old man, Marty? Nows we all hurting about your mom. You act like your father, my best friend.

Now, do not shut us out. You will regret that Marty."

"Your right. Hell. Thank you. Do not be sneaking upon my Aunt Paula, ok Able Sable," Marty says back with a grin. "She gets scared."

The next day Marty starts his new job along with Matthew. After work the twins track down their father who has been in prison. They pay his bail. Janella waits outside.

"Thanks for everything Janella. I could not have gone through this period in my life without you, dear," says Marty.

"I love you Marty and I admit that now. Thanks for saying it to me," she responds. Matthew begins to shed a tear.

"Okay, I did switch the tests scores, I mean you got an A Marty, I switched our names."

"What?" Marty and Janella begin laughing.

"I already knew, Matthew," says Marty.

Moral: A true friend loves all the time and is a brother born for distress, a proverb.

The Snail and the Pink Watch

A long time ago there laid a dog constantly chained to a meter in front of this brick house. Little did we know he was a good dog because when he frowned everybody saw it as scowling? The only time he went into the house was during rainy weather.

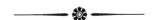

When it rained the snails came from it seems thin air. Most had hard shells. Perhaps they were blown in a certain direction by the rain they really are so slow.

So, one day a little girl whose favorite color is pink picked it up and put it on her watch.

"Nice pink watch," said the snail as his heart bounced to the tick-tock!

"You can talk," said the little girl.

"Yes. Is your favorite color pink?"

"No."

"You could have fooled somebody little bit."

Walking home from school alone every day gave the little girl an opportunity to exercise. Yet, when she got home from school she was so tired that she decided to nap.

"The little girl was putting her watch on the window sill, and taking off her heavy book bag, watching the snail who stayed on the watch looking out the window.

"Honey, good to have you home again, shouted the little girl's mother and father.

"I am resting/' she responds.

A throw rug in the middle of the floor, her square was a little resting place.

The little girl's book bag contained a science book.

The snail jumped back because she thought the snail was about to jump out the window.

"Dangerous, do not do that/' she said.

"You are my best friend. I know you miss your old teachers who were there for you but you can make new friends starting with me. Your teacher Ms. Stager told me to tell you she knew your laugh warmed her heart. May I sit next to you? Ms. Stager would want you to grow up. Her children are on the honor roll and she is very busy."

The next day the sun came out.

"How many colors do you see little girl?"

"I think one but the heat helps me coordinate a my visual art."

The snail kisses the little girl's hand because her skin is gold.

People will step on snails and will not notice them even if they are in a pack like coloring crayons. The little girl has dreamed of cooking like a chef but it's hot in autumn/ fall. To them art is for the shattered at heart but they enjoyed looking at art because this made them hungry like an end to a means safely.

I am going to call you rainbow girl for you are going places thinking critically. Now after school, put me down off this watch and you will study hard. You may go to the park."

"Leave you outside?"

The little girl with the pink outfit is more positive and sees how she was wanted.

Moral: You are not alone in the world. The earth is filled up with HIS loyal love. So stop acting like you are alone.

Separate and Friendly–Is it Possible? : Part 1

"Mommy am I better than Desiree?" asks Sarah Bergen. The Desiree she refers to is a red boned little girl. Her parents are black male and a white female. It is the 1890's.

Rutherford B. Hayes was a "staunch abolitionists" (Wikipedia) during 1877-1881 while he was President of the United States of America. So perhaps Desiree's parents felt it was okay to get married. But dear I do not think it is right," Mrs. Bergen responds.

Meanwhile Mr. Bergen is in another room listening.

"I don't either."
"Do you know she told me she got brushed by a brick that came through the window on the first day of school, Mommy? Mama, you did it didn't you, "a grimacing Sarah.

"Yes I did! So they moved up North and it will be better for them now. Although you should not do it because I did, Sarah."

"The things you say are a reflection of your soul," Mr. Bergen chimes in. Did you know your family lived on donations from the church Mr. Chung gambled his citizenship and won- a lot. He had too.

"Stop it, no! Are you saying I am evil altogether? I hope you are not saying that," says Mrs. Bergen.

"Mr. Chung was going to be escorted out the country until he was forced to fight for the lame country too young to be not getting along. Prejudice forced him to be philanthropically and not cynical. Sarah was my former bosses Auntie's name. She was not prejudice."

"Daddy, I want to be happy," says Sarah.

"I believe in equality daughter. Mr. Bergen pauses and looks to the side. In fact, we are moving up north so we may apologize to the Matthews and Desiree. At least for the summer."

"Here is your newspaper Hinny/' says Mrs. Bergen. Her first name is
Ariel.

"I will apologize so we can come back to the south eventually."

"Open your mind before you open your heart Ariel," replies Mr.
Bergen to the latter comment.

Moral: Self- explanatory

Separate and Friendly: Part 2

The Bergen family keeps their house well.

Sarah would like to visit her father's career to study fire in the tavern. Already she has learned how to make a spark using twigs. Her mother does not let her cook meals yet. Yet, the fire in Mr. Bergen's store blazes very high and the whole entire bar gets warm.

The tide of racism might linger a bit. You can change laws, not hearts.

Nonetheless, meetings on a judicial level include just white men voting.

Mrs. Bergen starts to get preoccupied in the politics of it all. That is when she learns that you reap what you sow.

Sarah starts getting bullied in class. Sarah does her best not to reply in an angry manner to the girl who lifts her nose at her in her eyes.

"It takes one to know one No one likes your family anymore Sarah," says the bully. (((Since what your mama did to Desiree."

"She was just a kid," says Sarah superficially. I do not know why my mother did that."

"Right! To me you are a phony bologna."

"We are going to visit them."

"I hope your wagon breaks down on your way back from the north."

"If it does we will just have to build a road. You do not think you can talk to me any kind of way, do you? Where is your white pride?"

"Racism is a hungry cat, Sarah remember that."

During the Bergen family's sojourn to the north they actually lose a horse frightened by a beehive. Camping along the way, and eating snacks nobody chats. This is just a duty visit. There are soldiers on the border of each state.

"Put that old man on the horse for a while, "the officer says about Mr.

Bergen.

Then the Bergen family realizes he is a friend.

Moral: I think African Americans worry too much about racism. We already have black history month. When you keep on talking about racism it separates and every race needs to be strong. There is good and bad in every culture.

Where Cats Bow

Once upon a time there was a cat named Demetrius who liked to play bowling ball. Demetrius was orange and had white spots. The spot in front of his nose was bear skinned because once he fought with a dog named Ruffin.

Each other day Demetrius wept at the corner of the bowling alley at 7pm at night. There he was in the middle of 7 cats who circled him. All these latter cats had owners but not Demetrius. So they loved him.

Moral of the story: To onlookers these cats look conspicuous but they have feelings and think and can teach us how to befriend someone.

Three Dogs Down

Once upon a time there was a pet store. A dog named Petunia had a puppy.

Next the puppy says to the other dog how much he looks up to her.
That she too is a good mom.

Three people come into the pet store but there are only two puppies.
The other puppy says to the Mommy's "I think he is hysterical."

I think you are schizophrenic he says in reply. He bit the store owner.

Moral: Nice words bring out the best in others while the opposite is true.

Finding a Bubbling Creek

"So, I am getting married mom and I hope you will attend," says Donnie.

"No. I cannot. Must not! I think you are making a mistake."

"Why is that?"

"I do not want it to work out and you prove me wrong!"

"It takes one to know one," his fiancee Cara starts to say in her mind.

A tear rolls down her cheek.

"Let us go Cara," says Donnie.

On the elevator down the coop- building corridor is an elevator. Donnie and Cara smooch the entire way.

"Get a hotel, you people/' says his father whom catches his son and fiance smooching.

"And my parents went on to live happily ever after and then they of course gave birth to me," says Samantha.

"Wow, that was one sad story," mocks Timmy.

"Thank you," says the college Professor.

In reality, Timmy has a crush on Samantha but she does not know it.

Samantha gets a job at the school library to help pay for her tuition in a work-study program. Timmy sees her there and apologizes for mocking her during class.

"It was really deep; I get antsy some of the time on a subject like abuse, Samantha."

"You are forgiven," answers Samantha.

"Now, put this book back for me librarian."

Timmy laughs and leaves a book on the library table. Samantha blows her breath.

The next day Fabiola, who is Samantha's dorm roommate they get to know one another better. Their room is large with a bunkbed. A week after that Timmy calls the room.

"Hi my name is Fabiola."

"Hi Fabiola. I really called to invite your roommate to lunch with me. My name is Timmy."

"Enchanting! Sorry I will take a message for her.

The phones are hanged up.

"This date has two parts, then babe," says Samantha.

"You want to show me a middle class lifestyle, but, I am poor for now. May I go first?"

I will take you to Chelsea for a philly cheese steak on the cart. There are plenty of those, ok?"

The two young lads Timmy with Samantha leading the way buy sandwiches then; they hop on the subway/train system in New York City obviously. Their next stop is in the Bronx the poorest county in America last time I checked. On 16th street is a Jamaican restaurant w/ the best coco bread, and a video shop.

"Fabiola is home, she can watch the movie with us?" Samantha asked Timmy.

"Or we can leave the door open, babe. Thank you for tonight, Samantha."

The following day is a Sunday. Samantha meets Timmy. He is waiting for her with a royal blue PT Cruiser. She is wearing black leggings and a sponge like Nautica blouse. Timmy opens the door.

"What a gentlemen you are, my boyfriend,"

After the couple eats at I HOP they go for a walk in Botanical Gardens.

"You see that bubbling creek, Samantha babe.

"Yes."

"No one knows where it began or how much it will run over and it's kind of like our love. Let us pray our cup runs over with joy and wine, when we're of age of course. I love you. May I kiss you?"

"Not yet," Timmy.

The couple refrains from touching early in their relationship this allows them to share ideas on parenting one day down the line. Soon Samantha's father dies and she goes home to bury him. Timmy misses her at school and when she comes back to school she looks different.

"Timmy, my father flew away. I mean, I know he was really sick," she starts crying hysterically.

"Do you know Samantha babe why I admire you. It is because of your character and your strength." And I am here for you. I love you so much.

Will you marry me?"

"Yes, yes ... kiss me now like we were birds," says Samantha.

The wedding is a blast. Fabiola was a bridesmaid.

Dionne is Timmy's best friend.

Moral: No one has a monopoly of problems. When it rains blessings, it pours.

What is Schizoaffective?

A short story for self-help and awareness

I could just tell you about me because it could be helpful- but the real me. The girl Daddy saw when I was walking towards him at 20 years old and looking more like me. I cannot say 18 hospitalizations real easy on a family because it is not. That is how many you want to have in 18 years not 12. Just to be sure, not sorry.

Some of this story is truth. However due to the nature of schizoaffective you will be happy to know that some of this story is fantasy- like. Although sometimes I wish it was not.

Chapter 1

Beating the odds

There are 9 different symptoms of schizoaffective. Hearing voices, racing thoughts, forgetting who you are and just plain forgetfulness, there is sexual presuming, loss of self-worth, paranoia, ideas that are peculiar, and boredom. Any one of the combinations would make one feel demonized. I am pretty sure some Salem witches were just mentally ill. "People also ask" which is a feature of google chrome their questions that have no inexperience in which a *human being* feels when they're going through facts of the explanation.

Grandma Inez was a little Riddles. "I like to spin circles around people," she told me as we watched a family friendly teenage girl flick called The Sisterhood of the Traveling Pants. "I want people to think I am intelligent." This was Grandmas reason. She was beautiful and she ran with the Black panthers. I read a book about the Black Panthers they are different races.

One of their accomplishments include a New York railroad union, they went to college and started programs.

I learned from Grandma that schizoaffective is not from both parents.

Grandma blessed me to be a respected member of the hood. For a minute, it worked. I had a boyfriend named Jesse whose family is well known in the neighborhood. His mom was a wife and politician. She and her sister are missionaries at a local church. But church is not for me. I prefer the structure and zeal of Jehovah's Witnesses. There is love and trust there. During the time before I left to go with Jesse, I was hopeful. Everyday 24/7.

They warn us about promiscuity at the partial hospitalizations courses too. I am fortunate• to be alive. During the time when I was not with the Lord I became addicted to prescription medication and attempted suicide. It was the Macartha Park River where nobody makes it out alive. The river is dark and murky but if God looks after fools…

The life expectancy for women with schizoaffective is over 17 years less than the average and 14 years for men. There is no one in the world that looks like you. If you are a twin with the illness who here knows your unique personality. I like to spend time with other mature people to gain perspective like I did with Grandma. When she died I went ballistic. I actually started dancing before crying. One of my moves was stolen and used in a dance about dancing rivalries. It was in the air. So low self-esteem comes because people underestimate what I can accomplish. Some of my relationships I was used. A doctor had sex with me against my will and I was a virgin. He treated me knowing he was like an executive and me a promiscuous secretary. He then left his "city lab" shirt on my bed. I tried to fight when although I was drugged. So my self- esteem relates to God's blessing. Spirituality is a must I guess I keep going on too because Daddy said I could accomplish anything I put my mind to. But that was before my diagnosis.

Chapter 2

My boyfriend

I have relationship episodes. My worst fear is not getting married but due to the illness because I love the wrong men. I am straight. But Dennis we hit it off quickly. He is a white male about 5' 9", a beautiful soul. He got his elbow shaved by a train. But when we were in the Homeless Shelter, I sat on his lap during dinner because there were not enough chairs. He kissed me after our first day out together. We went shopping and played horseshoes of a sort. We were supportive but I do not like one way he spends his free time. I still love him ... When I moved we lost contact and although he does not write me back or call I am good for catching up with him 2,900 miles away to go visit which is just unreasonable my case worker says. I have a big heart and I want Dennis to know the real me. Because I was sympathetic when I was with him. I told him my name is Christine and that I was 10 years older and that I have HIV. He still wanted to know me. I just forgot who I am, who my parents are. For years I did not know my mom. That was an episode. Imagine having a conversation with a woman who you know is familiar but insists on telling you how to do things. It was aggravating and I got an ulcer.

So far I have brought up 9 symptoms of schizoaffective. To explain it in further detail here is the first one- delusions. Delusions are a false belief that one cherishes despite having no evidence that it is true. This can happen because my racing thoughts are trying to connect what I know. The only problem we have with this symptom is that the stigma does not allow for talent. Talented people do not think like the majority although we can understand them. We strive for excellence or superiority in our field. So delusions may sometimes be a misunderstanding or differing opinion.

I also brought up sexual nature because the anti- psychotic gives one a jerky feeling. So I used to find myself looking at a man I normally would not like just because I looked for a while. There is an obsessive component that follows behind being tired of the jerky movements.

Fourth- forgetting who you are. It can have you fantasize being someone you admire.

Fifth- feeling low self-esteem which can come about of feeling not understood because of your illness. It can also be associated with just being ill. I feel good and then physically, pain follows. Therefore, the right medicine is necessary. Naturally, I begin to associate feeling good about what I like with something bad. Searching for a good doctor can be difficult. Remember your spirituality.

Chapter 3

Finding Time for Myself

I get bored because the social security lady told me it would have been better for me financially if I did not work. Such comments make me feel like not working hard because it seems the government is designed for some people to be poor and stay poor. I have put myself through school/college by social security and became something. But, people with disabilities get the end of the stick. In courts and in college applications I have faced prejudice. If I did not work I would be getting a government hand-out. Some people feel I am. But basically all I get is food stamps and people I will have you know have food stamps in lower Manhattan on the first of the month. It could mean early retirement.

I get bored not working. Therefore I have been working on getting work for the third time. I succeeded twice then dropped out due to laziness.

I guess something easy for me will be good.

My case worker helps pay part of my rent her and her company but it comes at a price. Enforced are home visits so I *must* be home sometimes.

Basically if I am not careful my life encompasses mostly appointments, food shopping and cooking, eating, doing cleaning and that is it. Hence I look for ways to enjoy life to the fullest extent. Reading, writing, playing games with a friend, watching good movies on my phone require ingenuity. I used to have a photography hobby. I like to travel and write about that. Going out to parks and theatres is fun. The more I am entertained my creative brain is stimulated. I have gone to Titanic and the Dead Sea Scrolls exhibit, Sesame Place with souvenirs, concerts, the Color Purple on Broadway, Aida, the White House, museums, Dorney Park, and many other places. Boredom means I am going through an episode. This too shall pass.

Chapter 4

Disturbia

It all started on a stormy day in the end of April. I was leaving my good friends like in another box. I felt like exploring science. I wondered about plasma because it is in the sun and in the T.V. and in the human body. So I wonder if I could, at the right setting of the moon, put a man I would marry on my hip. He had to be someone younger than me but a teenager because I was 16 at the time. I wanted to help him get out of his own lonely way, help him. I saw words on my hip in a bubble like smoke. It is like I got what I wished for but everyone felt I was hearing voices and was paranoid. Electrons and protons combine. That is as bad as my disturbia went.

Most people with mental illness are not harmful like I am not. Except I have tried harming myself. One time I thought I was getting even with my
Mom and would take impulsively too many of the pills she had prescribed by the doctor for me. The second time I was afraid to let the ice in my heart melt by going to a dance with and it turns out- the truest friends.

The third time I was depressed because I thought I could not have another baby because it was taking a long time. However, a baby deserves two parents married: a Mommy and a Daddy. Each parent supplies something their inheritance would need. It is simple to say food and money are involved with taking care of their baby. But a Father for example his example can teach children to have self-esteem for their name, courage in the face of difficulty and getting work done completely. Mommy is the nurturer. She imparts qualities such as patience, loyalty and love, fairness and others through love and consistency for her mate.

Sometimes I would assume that hearing voices which only happens to some sufferers, makes one crazy. But many sufferers have found that the adage "if you can't beat them, join them" has bode well in subduing voices. I find that voices can even work for you like a cuckoo clock, alerting you to a job well done and alarming you when you need not hear it. Like my phobias are attuned to my brain and voices on occasion will annoy me about those phobias. I will not mention what those phobias are.

Chapter 5

Calm after the Storm

My brain has a defiency but my problems are relatable and we can still put ourselves in others shoes. I hate it when someone holds back from telling me her problem because she thinks mine are too much for one to handle. Holding back may seem like the sympathetic thing to do but it robs me of making you my close friend. Friends are not meant to be used for different functions of one individual either. That was my mistake in befriending somebody in my past. She said all types of weird things like the above, did not know anything about true love.

What makes me normal is that I do not cry often now only like at funerals and baptisms and weddings, maybe even baby showers. I know I will have a baby one day. I have a desire to build a family which is a normal desire. I like a clean home, good food and I bleed if you scratch me. Please do not scratch me. I need friends. I need love. I think about college and a long day at work feels satisfying. When I was in college I averaged an A not an A- or A+ right in the middle. I am not perfect. I have made mistakes in my life that I am learning from every day. There are certain unique skills I may have mastered like Sudoku. I can solve a puzzle in 12 minutes. I am a writer of plays, movies, poems, stories and now this self-help excerpt. I have nieces. I have been in weddings. I have been beaten up. I have gone to prison. I have been shot at. I have fallen in love. I feel I can teach because as the adage goes /(been there, done that".

I have one wish too. That Beyonce pays me for giving Destiny's Child the title "Cater 2 U". I met Kelly Rowland when I worked for Whole Foods Market 59st Columbus Circle.

Now you know what Schizoaffective is really like.

Psychosis in any state is triggered by a negative event in one's life.
Mine has a long history. Basically, I learned to take myself and people therefore for granted

which led me to chronic loneliness. And after I was raped, I started taking psychotropic medicine. One doctor thought I may have some of his (the violator) personality because he was bi-polar. I have faced a lot of jealousy. These combined caused me to eat my sorrows so I can also defend myself and look less attractive. If God could talk to me right now I think he would say 111 am happy about your progress, Tabitha." I do not wear labels anymore. I do not blame anyone in particular for my troubles. The best revenge is to live well. The point is I am concerned about myself because that is my greatest insurance.

If experience is a teacher than I have learned not to be too hard on myself, to seize the day (carpe diem) and to please myself when I feel the crave. Life is too short to keep bad friends. Now, you cannot choose your family. Fight and pray is my motto. I don't know how to best explain that I'm here. If I got an opportunity to give my 16 year old self advice I would first say do not be modest with love- there is no age limit.

Secondly, do not be afraid to complain because there is a way to do it right. You let problems cause you to blow the rooftop.

Third, I guess that is it until another rainy day.

Fourth, do one thing and stick to it. Don't settle for less. If I had these points in my heart when I met Neyo, Julia Stiles, Eminem, Justin Beiber, Mariah Carey, Jamie Foxx, Simon Cowell and Timberland in California I would have stood toe to toe with them. If there is one thing I would like everyone to know is that we're all glorious.

Conclusion

I have two other mottos: (1) Give everything you do 100%. (2) I used to tell my first I will not let anyone take the blame for my sins.

I have written this excerpt because there was only one blog on managing Schizoaffective Disorder when I was diagnosed with the illness. Awareness is lacking. The National Alliance on Mental Illness (NAMI) offers these suggestions for sufferers: Pinpoint your stressors and triggers to prevent feeling excessively tired or end up in crisis. It could be "people, places, jobs, or even holidays" (website for NAMI) that trigger your symptoms. And avoid drugs and alcohol even when somebody promises to pick you up. Establish a routine and form healthy relationships. Yes, getting active is a plus. Have someone there when you need down time. You may need a therapist. You're eventually going to be able to work.

What patients go through is difficult for everyone. I may not remember my fellow patients by name. Nevertheless it was on the ward floor I learned so many lessons and my "brains physiology, and perhaps even its structure" was altered by the visits to the wards, (the healing power of gardens, New York Times- Olive Sacks journalist.)

I was so young my first hospitalization and yet I became addicted when away from the wards. People pity you when you are really young and going through a hard time. It changed a lot as I entered my thirties. The food in psych wards are very good and the plates generally full. But tying people down is wrong. It is tearful to look at.

I learned 3 lessons: The outdoors should be pleasant if they're not, there is a trigger about to happen. Everybody denies they have a mental problem. It is not for the reason you might think- the stigma. Not really.

It's because of their family's reputation. Finally, mentally ill people are dominantly religious and have the gentlest hearts.

All it takes is having a goal on healing and a doctor to believe in that goal.

Had to be the One

I was born with Narcolepsy bouts of tiredness. The illness is uncomfortable. At the family picnic my cousin played a trick on me because I went to sleep. I would like to thank the relative whom I inherited Narcolepsy from.

I remember the time, I was in gym class. Everybody was climbing the rope. My turn came. I stood up, energetically, made it over, put my hands to the rope, and without fear I fell asleep. By the time I was awakened class was over and I sustained a little knot on my eyebrow.

My name is Nia and I have Narcolepsy.

Moral: Think about the persons in the world who have it worse than you. You will have faith and feel better.

The Lighthouse Keeper

"You are my favorite daughter, alright, Kilars, because I know your brother and sister are best friends," said Missy Kilars mom.

"I am not jealous Mom," said Kilars.

Welcome to Rhode Island where there lives a family of five: Darmy is the Father, Tanya Mom, Kilars the oldest child, Pip the son, and Dolores the youngest daughter.

Darmy owns a lighthouse that alerts passing ships of danger. One Saturday morning while Darmy was working and Tanya was working Kilars was almost raped by a neighbor who knew the family well. Kilars told on him and that man went to jail.

Still, at times Kilars seems to get agitated without cause. In High school now Dolores picked up ceramics class and she taught Kilars how to make a mask. As the ships went by everyday Kilars would put on the mask and standing in between the light for the ships and she kept a pumpkin with a candle I it.

"What do you want from me?" asked Kilars when she was caught. She went on to explain: "Unless the face of the pumpkin is carved out you do not know it was good for something," she whimpered.

"Hunny, your flashbacks have touched my heart and I am truly sorry. Your Father and I were ashamed at what you went through. We are all going to get pass this together. Kilars was hugged by her parents.

Moral: You cannot trust everybody. Rape whether it is a boy or girl victim is wrong. Get help for major depression.

Her Story

It was like the weight came off her no.2 pencil as she wrote. Darling always looked serious and no one bothered her. Her pudgy, lined, fudge wrapped fingers looked like Ninja Turtle fingers, if you would ask the class.

Darling used to sit in the corner by the window, her body a 90 degree angle in the chair. She wrote, and wrote, and wrote some more.

Was it about romance, action packed drama, nobody knows. Except when she got up, her eyes lost their puffiness, there were no bags under her eyes. Today, we have learned about the dirt she took off, and all the sadness work on a no.2 pencil and loose-leaf paper.

The End

Billy Sunshine

"Mama, why is it dark at night outside and light in the daytime?" asks a scrambling little Billy at bedtime.

Rose tucked Billy into his full size comforter bed cover and kissed him on the forehead.

"Billy, I am going to tell you a story. When I was your age, my mother told me the same story. So I consider it a privilege to be able to tell the story to you.

"Mrs. Sun worked very hard. Although she got tired this helped the flowers to grow and a good time for the children to play. Mrs. Sun smiled because she was helping and that she knew she could help. But one day Mr.
Moon found her crying.

"What is it?" says Mr. Moon.

"Mr. Moon I worked hard to help my family, for the lilies to grow, and the children human to play outside, but... I do not have time to spend with my own family."

Mr. Moon says "There, there Mrs. Sun I have an idea. Let's share your work hours. You will shine for half the day and I will shine the rest of the time.
Mrs. Sun smiled brightly.

"I hate to see you crying," says Mr. Moon.

"Thank you so much."

Billy yawned and shut his eyes again.

"Goodnight my sunshine," says Rosa, You'll work hard tomorrow.

Moral: Play hard and work hard and rest hard.

How the Porcupine Got It's Quills

There was a 10 year old porcupine named Tingle. He had no quills. This would soon change. In winter, Tingle traveled with his Grandma and Grandpa to a warmer climate. They went through the forest of Kansas, the dessert of New Mexico, and went into Arizona. On the rocks there was a fox that scared Tingle soo much when he saw her that he shook, and let out a scream and all his hair stood on its ends! Grandma and Grandpa were so proud of Tingle. He scared the fox.

Moral: And that is how the Porcupine came to have quills.

Description of a Superhero

I have layers of characteristics. My four superpowers each leave me
45 degrees cold when I use it. I reveal what is within man 50 percent goodness and 50 percent badness. I am dainty. I am edgy. I feel words on my hips. I am like a rock star considered a god to some. Do I view myself as one- nope! That is what makes me so super! Super son is my estranged brother. The villain on Superman 4. You may never want to fall in love after meeting. No trickery is involved in my game. Everybody loves my 30 friends. And I am super sun the female one.

Moral: You have weakness but you may use them to your advantage if you are smart.

"An Hour to Begin"

Tara does not know why she likes to hear female singers over male singers now as an adult. Tara cannot relate to celebrities. She uses the music to ignore her abusive relatives. They call her names.

"There is a rocking chair at home," Tara wonders about every time she is leaving her relatives.

At school where she works her has a duty- clean the turtle poop out of his water. She is thinking of assigning the duty to a student.

Everyday seems like she has to find a cure for her robotic behavior her relatives have wounded her so bad.

You may be able to tell Tara is suffering because she is always cleaning something and that is what she feels about herself and what she needs others to see.

"If you were able to describe the bracelet that was stolen, was it valuable?" Tara's friend the guidance counselor asks her.

"I remember now where I lost it. I am so sorry for bugging you." One day at school Tara gave the assignment to write a skit at each table about Egyptian rulers and gods.

The children ate Egyptian dates and made masks and costumes. It is not about what you believe in as much we all learn at the same time, in the same way.

Moral: You can learn from history and poor examples in your life.

Donovan and the Three Dogs

A long, long time ago there was a starry eyed dog named Donovan. Donovan was a Shitzu my favorite dog. He lived on a ranch with cows and horses.

It was a rainy day on the ranch and Donovan was indoors with his Master. The horses, *cows,* chicken and spider heard some gossip which they were offended by. The neighboring dogs felt Donovan was too talkative and young and stupid so they planned to pick a fight with him. Three against one.

So on the dawn of the day it was just partially cloudy and as the three approached the chicken cackled as loud as possible, the cow kicked his hind legs and it sounded like he was saying move instead of moo. The pig snorted and they carried on scaring the dogs.

See, the spider was thankful Donovan avoided sweeping her webs, the cows we never allow children to hop on, the horses were still wild and the pigs, well, enjoyed getting in the mud like Donovan.

Moral: No kindness no matter how small ever goes forgotten.

A Mothers Smile

At 7am Pauline rolls over in bed just slightly but her husband hears the alarm too and tells Pauline to wait because he will shut it off. It is a weekday, their sons' first day at Kindergarten in a private school. Pauline feels her husband's hand on her shoulder and she stops dreaming. She can only dream because her husband loves her. Pauline wakes up smiling because she thought about a buffet that makes only chicken in her dreams.

Apparently their sons' alarm clock went off by the fact he stands in front of the parent's door.

"Mommy I think I am sick," he says.

"I will talk to him," says Pauline's husband.

"Champion shirt for you my son. You will be a good student and you have a likable personality. So there is nothing to be afraid of, alright?"

"Thanks Dad!" The son responds. Pauline's son goes to finish getting dressed.

"Look at you. You're just as handsome as you were ten years ago," says Pauline when her husband goes back.

Pauline is eyeing him. She is out of bed and she hugs him around his shoulders.

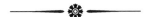

Two days passed officer. We have a good marriage and a son. How could my husband be missing but you promise to find him, promise me now, says Pauline at the local precent.

The officer promises.

Pauline's family lives in a double- decker house. She rushes home where her Asian friend is babysitting so she doses off on the bus too tired to think, to drive.

Was her husband kidnapped? Do they want a ransom? Pauline's husband works at Wall Street and she cries thinking he got a bonus and went on a trip with some other woman. Not trusting anyone anymore she pays her Asian friend at home and says she will never again need a babysitter.

"Your son is gifted and talented/' says the foreigner. Pauline nods. Her friend walks out at that.

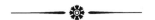

"AII day if possible, nobody will see you behind that mattress. My name is Jack sir. Do you like television?"

"Yes I do, says Pauline's husband. I know a soup kitchen in this city but you will have to walk around to City Hall. What is wrong with you? Try to clean up at the Native American museum or go to a shelter Jack. I miss my family, no, wait I cannot go home, looking my wife in the eyes and tell them I lost my job.

Pauline's husband is homeless now and his hair grows long and he is really scared. Yet, he hates the idea of becoming a statistic.

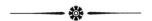

Talking to her out loud, "I wish I could make this decision with my man. Our son should be in a special private school." Pauline begins to cry.

A year goes by. Jack has found out he has enough change to cash in and buy a car for $800. Then, he leaves the street. So, he walks around thinking about how happy he is that he survived and all he can think about is watching a sports game with the guys at his relatives.

Pauline's husband goes into his home which has been paid off. It is in the middle of the day and nobody is home yet. He changes clothes and then falls asleep on the couch.

When Pauline comes in she senses somebody is in the house because of the kindred spirit.

"It's me Pauline! Do not shoot!"

"Dad, where have you been I missed you," says their son .

"I know you both no doubt thought I was dead."

"How could I think that about my husband?" Pauline smiles.

"I am so sorry; I need your help sweetie from you if I am going to get through this."

"Son, go do your homework," the parents say together.

They laughed.

"You Mr. have a lot of catching up to do with me, your son, the police and I would imagine your job."

"I lost my job I would have never given up that job. Do you understand? I tried to stay at a shelter looking for a future and I found out some of the meanest looking persons are homeless or so it appears. Or, it was probably in my mind. I was careful with my words and actions."

"My husband is home. I hear you. Maybe you need the Lord. Think about all the religions out there and choose one. I think you missed my cooking, you need to definitely shave, and invite everyone who you worried sick."

"The police knew where I was."

"Not the police in this rural town. Why? Why? Why?" He grabs her into his arm.

"Is it too late for me to apply for unemployment, Pauline?

"Well, we may have to fight for it. Our son is doing well, ok, but he is young, you get the drift? I never doubted. He did."

Making a Name

"I am alone. People point saying there are some birds above anything petty. The Butterfly wings are red, purple and orange. Their legs land on a traffic light and we hope it does not rain. My colors are yellow, brown, and white. Butterflies are beauty underestimated. Evening comes and I leave work. The Butterfly is on the second traffic light here in the south. Insects understand children need second chances. I know that about them because

I have eaten a few. Yet, I feel like feeding on the butterflies to get skinny.

On the opposite branch are the Pigeon and a Butterfly.

"Waking up is not encouraging/' says Pigeon to Mr. Butterfly. Pigeon eats.

"Humans are just as crazy/' begins the Butterfly. They schedule everything. They see Pigeons and chase you away but when I am on their shoulder they cannot feel a thing so do not walk, begin to run!"

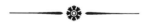

I like eating, it reminds me of my mother," Pigeon says to me the Bald
Eagle. Pigeon has 7 siblings.

"Every time the Pigeons meet they form a group and play in the water but one Pigeon does not I noticed. Perhaps she is pregnant. I cannot study birds because the field is off-limits. Still somehow I believe all flying creatures need human intervention to survive. Are the Pigeons running without a leader? My name is Ciao bane. I have five babies. All along I was doing well considering my unspecified mates. Everybody needs a family to give them the strength to keep silence on heated arguments. I eat different foods. If my family works at a Supermarket it is a bonus to me. Looking inward my family may write about where are all the birds. The simple fact that I am not anxious about my past, others are drawn to me as friends; and I love hunting to find out what is happening altogether. Bob is in College. If he does not shoot at me I will know why America loves my species.

Moral: Happiness comes from within. Animals are resilient but not human. Perhaps some native animals have learned that from Americans.

Heaven on the Mountaintop

As I read the note on the box: Don't open unless you're Ruthie. A spark of curiosity covers the sickening bewilderment I feel because my sister is dead. She wrote to me, Ruthie.

Dear Ruthie,
If the day passes by
And I don't get to see it
If the night comes in your heart
And I am not hear to know it
Know that we are a family
I am your best friend
I am your sister
And I love you indefinitely.
A tear rolls down her cheek.

The next morning Ruthie is bright and bushy tailed and asks her Mom if she could have a summer job like her sister would have to stay busy in good work. Ruthie's mother says yes. So does Ruthies Dad.

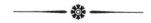

"Ok Ruthie, this is Fabi and this is Dion. She shows her the kid's pictures. They need to take a nap at 2:45- 3:45 every school day. Here is a copy of my keys. It is not easy being a Mom Ruthie. Do not rush!" says Mariana.

Ruthie smiles.

Fabi and Dion are being babysat. Ruthie makes them a peanut butter and jelly sandwich every day. They grow on Ruthie as if they realize what she is going through. They have compassion and are respectful.

One day on her way home, Ruthie sees a familiar sight of men hanging on the corner and she is happy she has a life.

The last day of her job Fabi and Dion who have moved to Tannersville, Pennsylvania huddle on the sides of Ruthie.

Way above the stable mountaintop

A miracle of peace comes and passes by

I want you both to be strong

Even when it is hard to say goodbye.

A tear rolls down her cheek.

Moral: The only guarantee in life is change. What does not kill you may make you strong.

Domino Effect-

(Non-fiction)

Citizens of all countries including America who are nationalistic imitate their leader or President. Frankly, it has been observed human beings are naturally born to have a role model. For many in the Bronx, it is Jesus from as far back as 2014. Yet even these people whom I have been privileged to meet will avoid a person who laments about trauma and prejudices quickly follow. Now, these factors are not particularly contributing to genocide today but accuracy better off with patience will help one to see; why Hitler was so bias toward two groups in particular. This story is non-fiction and were I to tell it right more Americans should visit the Washington D.C. Holocaust Museum.

On the game itself there are three ways of positioning your dominos. Noteworthy even a mere child can master the color coordination and the number of dots on the domino. There were children such as Anne Frank who was arrested and died during the famous and controversial Holocaust during World War II. Some people who feel a spiritual balance from a few being sacrificed in times of low mood and quiet promote the notion the Holocaust did not happen. But race comes up in every day huddles so we know that it's a lie. Jehovah's Witnesses who were killed by insolent men, dismembered too, are still the targets as they wrote to Hitler to stop and managed to stay neutral and innocently respect others. They do so by paying their taxes and educating themselves. 1/3 of them disappeared and their teenagers who were just making up their mind (on religion). None of the Jehovah's Witnesses were interviewed who remember the Holocaust in as were Jews. Hitler was an atheist *and* agnostic. I also believe Hitler was mentally undiagnosed unstable Dictator for the years he ruled.

Colonel George Stevens created the documentary of Anne Frank impressed by her story written in the concentration camps. He was healing. Hitler arose as a Dictator in 6 months upon the decline of Paul Von Hindenburg, but, he only won with 38% of a popular vote. No doubt the burning of Parliament hurt Germany who at that time soared in the field of Physics in the entire world. He blamed the Communist, even hunting its Dictatorships.

They paid.

Hitler's second in command created the idea of Gestapo. Paranoia gave birth to exaggeration and I am impartial. Anti-Semitism started with the boycotts by the government.

Where books were burned, his future stage opened and being alive at the time was as different as losing a personal friend. I think Hitler was hoping Jews were led to commit suicide but they do not do things like that.

On another day 25,000 books were burned as a purification of Germany's culture. While the influential march to the music people suffered a lack of knowledge and were put in the ghetto.

A full Jew had at first three Grandparents Jewish but if you were brandished in a relationship with a Jew I believe happiness could only come when you were working and preparing to meet up again.

Story books for kids taught obedience only to Hitler and racism.

Jews were hated more than blacks.

The mentally ill were murdered and the handicap sterilized.

As in the days of slavery, children of blacks were sterilized when born from an interracial relationship.

A Hollerith machine records kept information on concentration camps prisoners and sorted them by God only knows.

I am a person who loves peace as opposed to war but radical decisions on Veterans made the German environment hostile. Germany ignored the

Treaty of Versailles and many writers as well as the League of Nations were disposed to make Germany suffer greatly later. Once again, Jehovah's
Witnesses did not retaliate although their stuff was confiscated and they refused to say Hail Hitler, not one.

Homosexuals were persecuted because they did not sow German seed.
Basically, Hitler broke their belongings and taxed them for it.

The book of Esther was read aloud by Jewish people in groups. Esther is a Bible book which Jews disheartened by oppression could appreciate only at that time. Now, their studies mostly make up the Torah and traditional commands by their leaders.

Anyway, if you were chronically ill Hitler saw you in the hospital too much, you were useless and killed. These people all remembered by someone we hope because it happened...

During the Olympics when Jesse Owens won the relay races Hitler paid tribute to the black American since he was heartless and thought his country would dominate.
Remember Babi Yar which refers to all the Jews in Kiev Ukraine. Hitler managed to take over over there. In the concentration camps they were sent to their Typhoid Fever broke out on lice ridden bunks. The women's were shamefully shaven and raped on occasion.

Countries like Yugoslavia and Sweden also a man named Schindler were not struck to the heart over Hitler's antics. Kiaer Line was a boat emergency transfer spot Jews were moved by and hidden by a country away. A handful survived. Schindler transferred 1100 Jews. By combat, man to man, and with guns Yugoslavia helped Jews who revolutionary ideas were obviously natural. Certain reports state "the German problem" could have ended earlier if independent nations were more involved with what is fair.

Nuremberg refers to the trials America solved. On the site of Washington D.C's remodel of a camp at the Holocaust Museum, visitors around the world hide the face in disgust.

"I have sinned and my people has sinned against thy people and against thy self," said Martin Niemoller (1892-1984). He was disappointed in Hitler's regime even before he was arrested. He admits not liking some of the victims.

I wish what is right and wrong was not up to chance because the young people in those concentration camps were creative and now see life through black roses. "The German problem" is a sarcastic lack of charm on my part. The human who is resilient enough to live a day at a time with trauma owes the world nothing, I understand. So, do not act out and wreck less on bad days and you will have your share pick of wanting to morally so badly go to another place.

About The Author

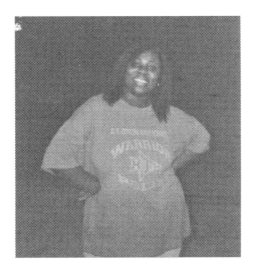

Tabitha never wrote about herself although she has about 100 pieces of literature to date. She has won a bookmark contest with a reading slogan. She has also won a children's book in High School. She writes from her heart, "It is hard to be real about anything else," she says. But her friends remember her as always cleaning up.

Printed in the United States
By Bookmasters